Chronic Faith

Chronic Faith

A believer's approach to chronic illness and pain

Allison J. Hampton

© 2012 by Allison J Hampton.   All rights reserved.

Published by Vantage Point Publishing
1833 N. Shadeland Ave
Indianapolis, IN 46219

No part of this publication may be reproduced or transmitted in any form or by any means, electronic or mechanical, including photocopy, or any information storage and retrieval system, without permission from the publisher. The only exception is a brief quotation in printed reviews.

Limit of Liability/Disclaimer of Warranty: While the publisher and author have used their best efforts in preparing this book, they make no representations or warranties with respect to the accuracy or completeness of the contents of this book and specifically disclaim any implied warranties of merchantability or facilities for a particular purpose. No warranty may be created or extended by any persons. The advice or strategies herein may not be suitable for your situation. You should consult with a professional where appropriate. Neither the publisher nor author should be liable for any loss of profit or any other incidental damages, including but not limited to special, consequential, or other damages.

This is a work of fiction. Names, characters, businesses, places, events and incidents are either the products of the author's imagination or used in a fictitious manner. Any resemblance to actual persons, living or dead, or actual events is purely coincidental.

ISBN 978-0-9883939-1-2

The publisher would appreciate notification where errors occur so that they may be corrected in subsequent printing and/or editions. Please send comments to the publisher by emailing to biz@amorousink.com

Printed in the United States of America

DEDICATION

Chronic Faith is dedicated to the memory of my mother, Martha Jean Hampton. Her character was legendary and her faith, boundless. Thank you, Mommy, for teaching me by example to believe beyond what I can see, to dream big and to walk in the expectation that God will fulfill all of His promises. Because of you, I know that faith is not a practice—it is a lifestyle. I love you.

ACKNOWLEDGEMENTS

I am grateful for God's faithfulness, and for His love that He has manifested through so many people.

To my family, I would be nothing without your constant support and encouragement. Thank you for your prayers and unconditional love. I love you.

To my friends, your selflessness and generosity have been a blessing. Your thoughtfulness will never be forgotten.

To every medical professional or associate who contributed in any way to my treatment and recovery, words could never be sufficient to express my gratitude. Your efforts are priceless to me. Thank you.

To everyone living with a chronic condition, and to all of the people that care about them, you inspired this book. I encourage you to never give up. Your life has value and it is worth the effort to find a way to live each day to the fullest. No matter how many times your symptoms resurface, allow your faith to show up just as consistently. Your faith must become as chronic as your diagnosis. That is how we win—by facing a chronic condition with chronic faith.

                          Expect Great Things,
                                  Alli

TABLE OF CONTENTS

Introduction		1
Chapter One	The Journey	3
Chapter Two	Acceptance	12
Chapter Three	From Sickness To Witness	19
Chapter Four	Where Is God?	29
Chapter Five	Misinterpretations of Faith	33
Chapter Six	Identity Theft	43
Chapter Seven	Tough Love	49
Chapter Eight	The Cost of Living	54
Chapter Nine	What If I Die?	58
Chapter Ten	The Mindset Of A Champion	64
Chapter Eleven	Chronic Faith	73
Appendix A: Simplifying Your Health Care Management		76
Appendix B: Your Medical History		77

INTRODUCTION

I am not a doctor. I never even played one on TV. But I am a warrior against chronic illness. In 2008, I was diagnosed with lupus. Then, in May of 2011, I was diagnosed with fibromyalgia. My life has not been the same since. More than anything else, however, I am a Believer. I believe in a kind and loving God. I believe that God has provided guidance for all of our situations and answers to all of our questions in the Bible. My name is Allison. You can call me Alli—all of my friends do.

I also believe that God gave doctors and scientists expanding knowledge of the human body so that they can help His people. But as helpful and effective as their information is, unless they have experienced your specific diagnosis, there are some things that they will never be able to tell you about your condition. They cannot address the emotional factor, or how deeply it will affect everyone in your life. When I was first diagnosed with lupus, I had as many questions as I had symptoms. I felt lost and confused— all at once, I had too much information *and* not enough. My emotions were all over the place, and I wasn't sure how to get them under control.

In 2010, I had a severe lupus flare—the worst I'd had up to that point. While I was hospitalized, one of my nurses, a lupus patient herself, talked to me about her personal experiences with lupus. She gave me the opportunity to be completely candid about my fears, concerns and frustrations. She did a lot to validate my emotional struggles and to give me hope. It was a significant turning point in my journey.

So, for others who are embarking on a new journey of chronic illness and/or pain, know that you are not alone. Be encouraged—the Bible says, "Better is the end of a thing than the beginning thereof…" (Ecclesiastes 7:8, KJV). When you are first diagnosed with something, you don't know what to expect and may have little to no concept of how to deal with your new situation. But the more you deal with the condition, the easier it will become to do so. I hope that by reading about what I have learned, you will feel less alone, less afraid, more hopeful and more at peace. This is not a how-to manual by any means, because our experiences, conditions, symptoms and circumstances will differ significantly. It is my hope, however, that your faith will propel you towards acceptance and a quality of life that is ultimately productive and full of joy.

Chapter One: THE JOURNEY

Life is good. Sure, there have been a few bumps in the road. You've had car trouble or an argument with a loved one. They canceled your favorite TV show. And the big ticket item you finally splurged on last month is on sale this week for 40% off! But these are the inconveniences of life that keep us sharp, cause us to employ our creativity and make us grateful for even the smallest blessings. Most of us have grown accustomed to dealing with day-to-day issues and even have an emergency plan for any minor crisis that may occur. If we are really fortunate, we have a support system in place that will encourage and help us through the occasional tragedy.

There is, however, no way to prepare for an ongoing disaster, so when that nagging pain or symptom finally becomes unbearable enough that you make an appointment with your doctor, and you are diagnosed with a chronic condition, it is perfectly reasonable to feel blind-sided. How is it that one sentence, a mere string of words, can change the entire course of the rest of your life? You are expected to calmly and maturely accept the fact that your body, as you know it, will never be the same again. You try desperately to navigate the barrage of terms, prescriptions, orders and warnings that are being hurled in your direction, barely understanding, much less remembering, what is being said. In fact, your hearing kind of short-circuited after you heard, "You have (fill in mind-numbing, terrifying diagnosis here). There are treatments to manage your symptoms, but, as of now, there is no cure."

This conversation kicks off what can be a long and difficult journey to a place called Acceptance. On this journey, you will make pit stops at several emotional locales. They are: Denial, Anger, Bargaining and Depression.

■■■

<u>DENIAL</u>: When first diagnosed, it is common to still expect to be able to function as usual. You plan your days as you always have—make commitments based on how you are used to feeling. It is difficult to understand why you are so drained mid-way through your to-do list. You are confused when six hours of sleep is no longer enough. And you are beyond frustrated every time you have to cancel your plans because you woke too up weak, sick or sore to leave the bed, much less, the house.

During this period, it is imperative that you are careful about what you say to yourself. Realize that there are a lot of things about your body that are going to be very different from now on. Resting when you are tired does not make you lazy. Declining an invitation doesn't make you anti-social. This kind of negative self-talk quickly becomes discouraging, because instead of motivating you to accomplish a goal, it causes you to push your body past its limits.

You will want to do the things you always have, and you will try to convince your body to cooperate with your mind. You are in denial. Trying to force your body to perform will only serve to frustrate and weaken you. Give yourself a break from unreasonable demands and focus on more realistic expectations. You will experience less stress and more success if you do. You may have convinced yourself and everyone else that you have superhero abilities, but it just might be time to retire the cape.

Furthermore, following your doctor's orders will be crucial. Your good days may be so good that you feel you don't need the medicine/therapy/treatments anymore. But your good days can become bad and your bad days may be worse very soon, if you neglect to do as prescribed. The adjustment will not happen overnight, but the sooner you can navigate your way out of Denial, the sooner you will be able to enjoy a better quality of life.

ANGER: So it's finally beginning to sink in. Your persisting symptoms are a constant reminder that your condition really is chronic. Translation: It's not going anywhere, so you're gonna have to get used to it. But you don't *want* to get used to it.

And now, you're just mad.

How is it possible that you are going to have to hurt or be sick, A LOT, for a really long time? How is it fair that you're going to have to take medicine and undergo treatments, quite possibly for the rest of your life? During this phase, every time you miss a wedding, birthday party, or concert of the year, you may find yourself seething, without even realizing why. Chronic pain and illness have a real tendency to cramp your style. You can't always eat what you want when you want. You can't always wear what you want because your weight fluctuates and the clothes don't fit properly, or the way something is cut is now very uncomfortable, and your skin is so sensitive that certain fabrics just hurt. Or maybe you are self-conscious about your body now and would never be caught in things you used to love to wear. Road trips and vacations are even hard because traveling takes a toll on you physically, plus it is hard to pack everything that you use at home to keep yourself reasonably comfortable. There are meds, canes, nebulizers, etc. to pack, appointments to re-schedule and the adjustments to new climates, time zones and surroundings.

Nothing is predictable anymore, and that can cause you to have to lean heavily on loved ones for support and assistance. Having to give up any measure of control and independence can be beyond frustrating. This frustration and anger can lead to stress that will exacerbate your condition and make your symptoms worse. It will also emphasize any negatives in your life and make everything a chore to deal with. Your life has changed, but you should still be able to enjoy it. You may have some limitations and losses, but you deserve to enjoy what you do have.

If you are ready to let go of the potential toxicity of your anger and embrace the happiness that awaits you, it is as easy as counting your blessings. *It's hard to be hateful when you're busy being grateful.* My mother always told me that no matter how bad things get, there will always be someone in worse shape who wishes they were in your shoes. When you feel anger rising, diffuse it with the thought of a loved one, a gift you have received, a hobby you enjoy or an experience you have had---something for which you are thankful.

Understand that anger is a natural and reasonable emotion. If you are blessed to have someone in your life who is a good sounding board for you, certainly take advantage of the opportunity to vent and blow off steam. Be careful, however, not to take out your aggression on innocent bystanders. The doctor who is trying unsuccessfully to regulate your meds and find a treatment that works is not to blame for your condition overall. A spouse who cannot understand your complaints or relate to your symptoms is probably not being insensitive on purpose. Try to keep these things in perspective. Focus on things that make you happy—things for which you are grateful. Smile at a stranger. Express love and appreciation to the people who are important to you. It will change the way you view your life and the challenges you will have to face.

BARGAINING: It seems impossible that so many changes could take place in your life all at once without your prior knowledge or consent. There must be some way to put things back the way they were. Is there something I did wrong to bring this upon myself? Is there something I should have been doing that I neglected to do? Often, friends and loved ones can unwittingly turn into miserable comforters (Job 16:2). In their efforts to make sense of your situation, they may suggest (sometimes without meaning to) that sickness or pain is somehow your fault (see Chapter 4).

Whatever the reason, we often think that we can negotiate our way out of a condition. But the reality is we can't make a deal or compromise—it isn't necessary. God does not desire that any of us should suffer. All that is good and perfect comes from Him. His desire is for us to prosper spiritually and be in health (III John

1:2). He allows pain and illness for a lot of reasons, but it is not for punishment or revenge.

Have you ever pledged that you would do something for God if He healed you? "I'll pay my tithes every week." "I'll teach that Sunday school class I refused to teach." "I'll go to Bible study faithfully." God is not moved by that type of bribery anyway. He knows that the only motivation for this change of heart is to convince Him to heal you.

Contrary to popular belief, you are probably not sick due to "lack of faith". Be comforted that God can, and *will*, heal you in His own time and His own way. Rather than trying to bargain with Him, your time and energy may be better invested in seeking His wisdom, strength, peace and grace to see you through what you are facing.

DEPRESSION: This last phase is characterized by a deep feeling of sadness and /or hopelessness that can lead to a loss of the will to do anything. It is during this phase that people tend to give up, withdraw themselves from friends and loved ones and even contemplate or attempt suicide.

It is logical to feel sad after you have withstood the other phases and are faced with the reality that your condition is not going to change. There is nothing left to do now but live with the symptoms and manage them as well as you can. In this stage, you are beyond emotions and reflect, with stark clarity, on all of the "never again's" and the "from now on's" that will so drastically impact the rest of your life.

Rather than considering this to be an ending, however, it may help to treat it as the beginning of a new phase. Instead of dwelling on what you can't fix, focus on the changes you can make to help you adapt. Enjoy the sense of accomplishment that comes from figuring out a new way to get something done. Challenge yourself to find as many ways as you can to feel better. For example, when something you ate makes you nauseous or an activity wears you out, put it on a mental or written list of things to avoid or limit. Next time, you can pat yourself on the back for being proactive enough to spare yourself some discomfort or inconvenience.

REALITY CHECK

There is nothing pleasant about being sick or in pain. But the whole experience is much more unpleasant when you dwell on the negative. Concentrate intently on your strengths and joys, however small. In time, the joy will become second nature and the negatives will take a backseat to happiness.

THE GRIEF CYCLE: Denial, Bargaining, Anger and Depression are pit stops en route to your destination, Acceptance. But these locales are also the five stages of grief examined in Dr. Elisabeth Kubler-Ross' Grief Cycle. Her research focused on sufferers of terminal illness, but I find these stages applicable to the experience of those being treated for chronic pain and illness. Though it is not always such a complete loss, it is certainly significant. Just like with any major loss (divorce, unemployment, foreclosure, etc.) a devastating emptiness and feeling of "lost-ness" can ensue and prove to be quite overwhelming.

Recognizing and identifying each stage can be helpful, because when you know the signs, you can counter the negative emotions with positive thoughts. It will be absolutely imperative that you learn how to talk to yourself. Faith still comes by hearing (Romans 10:17), and you will come to believe whatever you are told most often—even if you are the one talking. When you are tempted to say "I feel horrible", it may be more mentally productive for you to say "This is not my best day" or "Today has been especially challenging". This redirects your subconscious mind to days during which you felt better, which can encourage you, on a subliminal level, that better days are to be expected. Instead of saying "I hate feeling like this" or "Am I ever going to get better?", try to speak encouraging words to yourself. "I am grateful to be as well as I am" and "I am thankful that God has equipped me to handle this challenge". If you are having trouble producing (or believing) these affirmations when you need them most, it may help to have a few key scriptures memorized. "His grace is sufficient for me" (II Corinthians 12:9) and "The joy of the Lord is my strength" (Nehemiah 8:10) and "I am fearfully and wondrously made" (Psalm 139:14) or "I am more than a conqueror"(Romans 8:37). By rehearsing these scriptures, it reminds you that God's word is the ultimate truth, and you can believe it when nothing else is certain. What He has said carries more weight than your opinions or the doctor's prognosis. Peace, life and hope always reside in God's word. Your body takes its cues from your brain—that is why we must be transformed by the renewing of our minds (Romans 12:2). I can tell you that your body will not go any farther than you *believe* it can go. If you let yourself think you can't do anything, then you won't. If you choose to operate in God's strength instead of your own, then you can do what doctors call impossible. This brand of positivity becomes critical when moving into the last stage.

ACCEPTANCE: Let me start by saying that accepting your condition does not mean that you allow yourself to become enslaved by it. By accepting your new reality, you do not magically gain a license to make excuses not to live your life. Acceptance simply means that you will face pain and/or illness with a new determination, and by being aware of all of its implications, you can adjust to your situation in order to make your experience as positive as possible.

Acceptance is when you are able to face what is going on and make peace with it. Rather than fighting against it, you can work through it. Just like when a vehicle breaks down, ignoring it does not make the problem go away—it only allows the problem to become progressively worse. It cannot be fixed until you take it to the appropriate professional. Even if it still runs, the car won't run properly, which will cause greater damage over time. And, no, the mechanic may not use manufacturer-issued parts, but he can install parts that will make the vehicle run better.

Bottom Line: Acceptance simply means that you face the realities of your current condition so that you can create the best possible situation for your future.

Chapter Two: ACCEPTANCE

Acceptance, as it relates to chronic illness and pain, has to do with seeing your condition for what it is, coming to understand it, and learning how not to allow it to incapacitate you. Because your condition did not progress to this point overnight, it stands to reason that the process of accepting your circumstance will take time as well. It is reasonable that you might feel frustrated from time to time during this process. But understand that setbacks and stumbling blocks are not grounds for giving up. Acceptance tends to happen in three stages over time. There is no universal timeline in which you can expect this shift to take place. The stages are education, identification and adaptation.

EDUCATION

Athletic teams often prepare themselves for competition by studying films of their opponent's previous games. In doing so, they observe each player's strengths and weaknesses, responsibilities and tendencies. By learning what someone is likely to do, you empower yourself to be able to counter their usual moves, exploit their weaknesses and ultimately, upset their entire strategy.

Similarly, it is important for you to arm yourself with as much information as possible regarding your condition. At least initially, it may seem difficult to even face a condition with all of its inevitabilities and restrictions. It is scary to think of all the negatives and all of the possibilities associated. But, if you are honest with yourself, not knowing is even scarier.

My journey with lupus has been such an eye-opening experience, because I am constantly learning something new. For example, I recently learned that lupus can cause enlarged lymph nodes. As an isolated symptom, enlarged lymph nodes can be an indicator of a lot of things, or nothing at all. But the hematologist told me that there were no other indicators to suggest that the swelling was caused by anything other than lupus. It was a relief to have that information, because, had I skipped the appointment, I would still have been worried about having to face another condition. Moreover, you really benefit from knowing what you are facing by having advance knowledge as to how to avoid pain, address symptoms that arise intermittently, communicate with medical personnel and loved ones, and plan your days with maximum flexibility and minimum frustration.

Support groups and organizations can be very helpful in your efforts to learn more about your diagnosis. Your doctor's office should be able to provide you with contact information for foundations dedicated to researching your condition. Otherwise, an Internet search will quickly yield this information. Membership will likely include a periodic newsletter or e-mail blast, complete with information on upcoming events and gatherings, new legislation, medical breakthroughs and other noteworthy information. Another great source of information is Internet blogs. Finding a network of people who are having similar experiences can be very affirming. Sometimes it just helps to know that someone else knows what you are going through, that you are not imagining things and that someone else can identify with your issues. Some people can't relate, or find it hard to believe you because they are not used to you feeling or acting so differently. Some will even go into denial about your condition because they have trouble dealing with it emotionally. A strong support system can help you understand their reactions and give you insight as to how to effectively share information about your lifestyle changes with the people you care about.

Education decreases frustration. I encourage you to learn all you can about what is happening in your body. Apply the information and share it with others. The quality of your life will improve exponentially and you will experience less fear and more control.

IDENTIFICATION

Once you have gained an understanding about your condition—the basic facts, symptoms and research—then you can start looking for yourself within the documentation. For as many people as have been diagnosed with the same condition, there are that many different sets of circumstances, because everyone is affected differently by the same illness, will have different symptoms, be prescribed a different set of medications and have different side effects as a result. Every experience will be slightly different from someone else's and it will be most beneficial for you to find the symptoms and circumstances that most closely resemble your own.

The more that you see yourself in the cases that have been documented, the more you can learn from the mistakes, successes and discoveries of others. You will benefit from their creativity, validate your own experiences and share with others the things that you find helpful. I would caution you to not see yourself in *everyone's* issues. You will drive yourself crazy if you just wait for someone else's symptoms to occur in you. It may never happen. This identification process is only a part of your research—a fact-finding mission of sorts. Blogging can be very helpful, but no one else's account of their situation can be a how-to manual for how you should function through illness or pain. This information should help you transition into adaptation.

ADAPTATION

Reality can be difficult to accept, especially when it is beyond your control and when a situation is not of your own choosing. The good thing about acceptance is that once you are able to face something with total honesty, it is then that you can begin to use that knowledge you have gained to take back control and make your life better.

Do you find that certain chores tire you out a lot faster than they used to? There will be adjustments of many types that will enable you to accomplish daily tasks that you wouldn't normally be able to do, or simplify them so they are not nearly as taxing. It all comes down to doing things in a way that is easier and more manageable for you.   Break jobs into multiple phases, and rest in between. For example, if you are going to change your bed linens, rather than wear yourself out by trying to do it all at once, try it in stages: 1) Strip the bed. 2) Rest. 3) Put on the fitted sheet. 4) Rest. 5) Top sheet and bedspread. 6) Rest. 7) Pillowcases. It may take longer to complete the process, but it's worth it if you are not completely drained afterwards. Once you have that method down, then you can add other elements to the process. For example, when you get the fitted sheet on, take the pillowcases off while you rest. After the top sheet, sit down and put the new pillowcases on. Even your resting time becomes more productive that way.

Rest time is crucial—not just for big chores, but in general. Maybe you used to be able to function on three or four hours of sleep. Now, your body requires more rest to regroup and operate properly. Don't short-change yourself—give your body all of the tools it needs to be able to do all you will demand of it. Perhaps you haven't taken a nap since preschool. But if during the course of the day you find that you are physically dragging, give your body a moment to rest. If you can, consider taking a nap. If you are at work, spend part of your coffee break or lunch hour meditating on a scripture or inspirational song. Pray a prayer of thanksgiving. If power naps work for you, take fifteen minutes out and catch a few winks. But give your spirit time to rest and be refreshed by God's presence. Remember, *your body will let you know what it needs*. Maybe you don't want to take a break because you don't want to lose time. But if you don't give your body the rest it needs, you will wear down to the point that you will not be able to function at all. Then you will have to wait to accomplish anything until you can recuperate from rock bottom. A close friend of mine says it this way, "Give your body a chance to reboot, or it will hit 'CTRL-ALT-DEL' with no warning." He's right. If you do the things that will help you keep going, you will not end up starting from square one as often.

You will begin to notice challenges that start as soon as you wake up. Even getting your day started might not be as easy as it once was. It has been said that "time is not on your side". But that does not have to be the case. You can make adjustments so that time *can* work for you. If you are moving more slowly than you used to, don't put undue pressure on yourself to try to accomplish things in the amount of time that used to be sufficient. Rushing can make you forgetful, clumsy, irritable and frustrated. You may have to eliminate certain things from your routine or leave important items behind. That is a miserable way to start the day. Leave yourself plenty of time to do what needs to be done. Give yourself a small reward afterwards. Plan ahead as much as you possibly can. Do prep work in advance whenever you can. Load up the car the night before. Make meal preparations for several meals at once. Take time to organize things so that locating them later on is easier. When you simplify tasks and organize belongings, you day tends to go more smoothly. Easier days leave your mind and body freer to focus on dealing productively with your health issues.

If you have always been an active, independent person, you may be resistant to using the aids and devices that are designed to help you. For a long time, I was afraid that people would think I was being lazy if I used the motorized carts when I went shopping. But on several trips, I had to cut my list short and on others, I felt like I was going to pass out fifteen minutes after I entered the store. It didn't take long for me to realize that I'd rather let go of my pride than miss out on what I really want to do in life. I am no longer too vain to walk with a cane when I need to, because lying helplessly in the middle of the canned goods aisle, waiting for the paramedics, doesn't serve my vanity very well, either. Devices like grabbers, carriers, and medical alert systems can be very helpful to you, and can spare you a lot of pain, difficulty and unfortunate incidents while completing everyday tasks. You may look perfectly healthy to others, and at times, you may be criticized by those who are not familiar with your situation. Their judgmental remarks cannot be allowed to keep you from living your life in the most productive and safe manner possible. Sure, you look like the picture of health to those who have not spent any time with you, so they may think that you should not park in a handicapped space, board an airplane first or use a wheelchair or motorized scooter. But, do not let your pride cause you to suffer unnecessarily. Why put undue stress on your body, wear yourself out prematurely and forfeit the enjoyment and productivity that you deserve, when there are items designed to make tasks easier and more manageable? That is why they are there, right? Chronic pain and illness change your life, but life is still what *you* make it. Use your resources so that ultimately, you can make your life better.

Chapter Three: FROM SICKNESS TO WITNESS

No matter who you are or what you're doing, someone is watching you. "Even a child is known by his doings..." (Proverbs 26:11, KJV). I believe that two things reveal who you really are. One is how you behave under pressure, and the other is what you do when you think no one is paying attention.

Very few things in life are more stressful than pain and illness. It is often during those times that people tend to focus on themselves rather than others. The more we hurt, the less we tend to be concerned about the plights of others. No matter how compassionate you may be, the needs and wants, the pains and losses of others take a backseat to yours when you are dealing with your own suffering.

How is your personality affected when you don't feel well? Are you pleasant and considerate of others, despite your own discomfort? Or do you allow your pain and frustration to make you irritable? It's easy to let yourself believe that people should be understanding and sympathetic to your desire for attention and compassion. And although some people may be able to relate to what you are experiencing, how you are treated depends largely on how you treat others.

Any type of suffering can seemingly bring your world to a screeching halt. You may find yourself longing for a brief hiatus during which everything stops, in order to accommodate a very necessary adjustment period. If that's what you need, then by all means, take a step back. Even if you don't have the luxury of taking time off from work or sending the kids to Grandma's for a few days, make sure you set some time aside to spend alone. It can be tempting (and might seem easier) to just not think about your condition, but it is absolutely imperative that you take sufficient time to face head-on the realities and possibilities of your condition. In the long run, it is much more stressful to deal with changes and new developments in your health if you have not prepared yourself for them. Likewise, it becomes very draining to loved ones to be constantly blind-sided by the many curve balls that your illness can throw. Resist the urge to just "check out"—it doesn't help anyone.

Yes, it is scary to think about what might happen in the future—things you might have to give up, physical limitations, dietary restrictions and mandatory treatments. Let's not even talk about the changes to your appearance: hair loss, drastic weight gain/loss, scars, bruises, bumps, rashes and/or skin discoloration. Remember when you could eat salads, pork, ice cream, red meat and sweets without thinking about your blood pressure, blood sugar, cholesterol, lactose intolerance, or acid reflux? I admit, it is very inconvenient to have special food needs, especially if you plan to have a social life. But figuring out how to eat well can save you from embarrassing situations and keep you from missing important occasions. You can't figure out alternate plans, however, if you don't periodically examine your condition. Keeping a journal (even mentally) of your diet, activity and resting habits can reveal a wealth of knowledge to you and help you plan your days appropriately. Believe it or not, everything you do affects how you feel. And no matter how you try to deny it, how you feel greatly impacts how you act. People are usually somewhat aware of that fact, and will excuse testiness or irritability on occasion, but no matter how much you are going through, everyone still deserves to be treated with respect. As Believers, we should try to emulate Jesus, Who was loving and considerate of others, even as He suffered a cruel and gruesome death. As He gasped desperately for His final breath, His concern was for His mother's welfare, our forgiveness, and even a thief's redemption. Allow your personal discomfort to make you sensitive to the pain of others around you. Remember how it feels when someone who doesn't know what you are working through does not treat you with understanding and compassion. Who knows better than you that sometimes a smile is just a brave front for severe pain? Therefore, we should be careful to treat others with the compassion and kindness that we so often need.

PATIENCE FOR PATIENTS

Unfortunately, many patients lash out at medical personnel, often because they know that doctors and nurses understand their position and still have to take care of them, as opposed to family members or friends, who don't have to accept that kind of treatment. But these people who have dedicated their lives to meeting the needs of others take such undeserved abuse from many of their patients. Rather than add to that stress, why not make an effort to be the one who shows gratitude for their attention to your needs? You may be surprised by how far a "please" goes and how much of a blessing a simple "thank you" can be. When I was a child, I was taught that "please" and "thank you" were magic words. Who knew that the magic would still work after I grew up? Remember the story of the ten lepers that met Jesus (Luke 17:12-19)? He healed them and sent them on their way. Even though He had ministered to ten, only one returned to say "thank you". How will you be remembered when others read the parable that is your life?

My mother used to admonish me that if I wanted to understand someone, that I should walk a mile in their shoes. Think about a time when you did something nice for someone and they showed no appreciation whatsoever. Did you really want to do anything else for them? On the other hand, have you ever received a thank you note for something you didn't think was a big deal? That appreciation tends to make you more likely to want to do something for that person. It stands to reason, then, that a pleasant demeanor is more likely to be met with the same. After all, you can still catch more flies with honey than vinegar. At some point, you are going to need people, by virtue of the nature of the condition you face. Rather than alienating them, choose to be a blessing to those who may eventually be a blessing to you.

STOP STRESSING. BE A BLESSING.

You can't change your diagnosis. You can manage your symptoms, but it is highly unlikely that you can get rid of them completely. There are many things that are beyond your control when you deal with chronic pain and/or illness. And it becomes discouraging, at times, to have to give up the independence, spontaneity and comfort to which you are accustomed. But, once you face and accept your new parameters, you can begin to focus on your capabilities, your gifts, your strengths. It is reasonable to mourn the loss of your optimum health, but to dwell on it will lead to a painful and profound depression that will hold you hostage emotionally, if you allow it.

How do you turn a challenge into a positive experience? It starts simply with a decision. That may sound easier said than done, but if you have a habit of complaining or dwelling on how you feel life has "cheated" you, you will miss out on a lot of beauty, a lot of fun, and a lot of happiness. It has been said that the way to eliminate a bad habit is to adopt a good one to replace it. It is also said that if you want to create a new habit, you should practice it for 21 days. So, it is my suggestion that if you find yourself complaining about circumstances you cannot change, dwelling on your limitations or symptoms, or driving your loved ones crazy with your mood swings, that it might be time for a new habit. For the next 21 days, when someone asks you how you are doing, find something positive to say. When you begin feeling negative emotions rising, switch your thoughts to something you are grateful for. When your symptoms start to seem unbearable, do something kind for someone else. Send a "thinking of you" card or note to an elderly loved one. Compliment a perfect stranger. Give random inexpensive gifts for no reason at all. It is very difficult to feel down or depressed when you're focused on making someone else happy, and it is hard to complain when you are focused on what you have to be grateful for.

If you have had enough of dwelling on your problems, take some time to focus on the needs of others. Volunteer for a couple of hours. Serve lunch at a soup kitchen. Read to a sick, elderly or visually-impaired person. Babysit for a new mommy. Blessing someone else will *always* bless you.

WALKING OUT YOUR WITNESS

I have learned in recent months that people do watch you. And when you have physical issues, you are under even more scrutiny. You see, a lot of people guard their compassion closely, not wanting to worry about or accommodate others needlessly. But when it becomes apparent that your concerns are legitimate, it is easier for them to sympathize.

The true blessing comes, however, when you shift your focus from receiving sympathy to being a blessing to others. When you concentrate on what God has done for you, and dwell on the strength and abilities you still have, your faith walk becomes a witness. Others will see God's greatness in your life, because your conversation and actions will reflect your gratitude for the way He has taken care of you. When others see how faithful God has been to you, it will remind them that He will take care of them, too.

REALITY CHECK

Most people have no idea what you are going through. The average individual has an infrequent ache or pain, usually brought on by some identifiable cause. They may get the flu once or twice a year, or contract the occasional bug that's been "going around" at the office or the kids' school. They can actually get relief from their symptoms by taking over-the-counter medicine or the increasingly-less-common prescription antibiotic. So the concept of hurting all day or awakening to new symptoms each morning is completely foreign to most people. In fact, it is so difficult to fathom, that some are inclined to look at your myriad symptoms as little more than hypochondria.

At first, this will be very frustrating, and often, hurtful. The people you love and count on for support will act disappointed when you miss a gathering, or make you feel guilty for canceling an engagement. People who once respected you and applauded your work ethic and dependability may begin to regard you as a flake. Too often, people with chronic conditions will go to great lengths to avoid falling victim to these mistaken perceptions. They will make impossible demands on their bodies in order to live up to the expectations of others. They will push past their limitations to reassure others that they can still be counted on. Perhaps the greatest hurdle you will face is the blow that your condition can deliver to your self-esteem. A lot of one's identity is wrapped up in what they do. Isn't that how we describe people? "You know Katie—she's the one who directs the choir at church." Or, "Isn't Bob the one who's always working in his yard? It always looks like a magazine cover!"

When Katie starts dealing with the symptoms of her condition, and it becomes increasingly difficult for her to lead the choir rehearsal after working a full shift at her day job, she will probably continue , initially. She doesn't want to let anyone down. I mean, doesn't everyone have to make sacrifices for the ministry at some point?

Bob, too, might put pressure on himself to continue to do yard work despite his chronic pain. Sure—he will pay for it later by suffering for days after the grass has started to grow back and the flowers beds start to sprout new weeds. But what will the neighbors think if he hires someone to do it? Everyone else on the block does their own yard work.

People may think that you are lazy, seeking attention, or even that you think you are above your regular tasks. You can be sure, however, that they have never been in your position. If they had, they would recognize that there are some things that your body simply will not allow you to do. They just do not have the information or experience needed to be able to understand. Would you expect a second grade student to be able to do calculus? They cannot, because they lack information. Therefore, you cannot take it personally when others are not sympathetic to your situation. They simply lack information.

If someone's opinion is important to you, or may affect a significant area of your life, such as your employment, you may want to provide them with the information they need in order to be able to, at least, relate to what you're experiencing. At work, be as candid as the situation warrants--do not feel pressured to disclose more than makes you comfortable. HIPAA privacy provisions protect you from having to tell your employer the details of your condition. If you miss work, they can require you to provide documentation confirming that you are under a doctor's care. They are not, however, allowed to question you about the specifics of your condition or treatment. You may decide to share the basics with them so that they know what to expect. You might even ask your doctor to write a brief note explaining what you want your employer to know about your daily experience. Familiarize yourself with the Americans with Disabilities Act. There are laws that protect your right to work as long as you are able, and entitle you to reasonable accommodations. (For situation-specific advice, contact a legal professional.)

Your personal life is another matter altogether. Loved ones who are used to you playing a certain role will continue to have those expectations until they realize that you have new limitations. Search on-line and print out information detailing your condition and discuss it with those closest to you. Encourage them to join a support group for loved ones of chronic pain/illness patients.

For your toughest critic—yourself—support groups can be very helpful. It is very affirming to hear someone else describe exactly what you've been feeling. Check out Internet blogs pertaining to your condition—there is a sense of community and empowerment to be found amongst those who can relate to your experience.

Once you can give yourself permission to deal honestly with your physical demands, you will then be able to make the adjustments and accommodations that will almost immediately begin to improve your quality of life. **You are not obligated to justify any life changes you make.** When you go grocery shopping, remember that the motorized carts are there for customers with physical limitations. Instead of forcing yourself to walk through your local mega-mart and needing an ambulance by the time you get to the checkout, perhaps you should consider swallowing your pride. There is no shame in taking the assistance that was available to you at the front door. That's why it's there! Maybe, to others, you don't look like you need the cart. Of course, they haven't been with you at the doctor's office or the hospital, either—and they won't be accompanying you to the emergency room if your body can't handle the demands of your shopping excursion. In fact, you may never see them again. Don't fall victim to the judgment of strangers—they have some invisible issues, too. Everyone does.

■■■

Chapter Four: WHERE IS GOD?

I know that Christians traditionally are taught not to ask questions like this out loud, but it is an honest question, and I think it does more harm than good to avoid it. It cheapens our relationship with God to think that He is somehow too emotionally unstable or egocentric to face our issues and concerns with us. He created us with the capacity for a wide range of emotions, and He understands how we feel at any given time. His love for us is unconditional, and His compassion is unwavering. So, as we explore this question, let's commit to being as sincere with God as possible, and give Him an opening to speak to our hearts, even about the touchy subjects.

As Believers, I think we have certain expectations of how God should and will deal with us. We feel that because we have accepted Him as Lord of our lives, that He will be our Protector, Provider, Friend and Father. And it is true—our God is all of these things. But when bad things happen, it is human nature to question how God could allow them, and our faith becomes challenged.

So, guiltily, we go from emotion to emotion, conflicted by our circumstances and convicted by our beliefs. We want to trust God and testify that we know that He is in control. But when we are along with our thoughts, and yes, even our fears, there is a little voice in the back our minds that demands to know "Where is God?"

My chronic illness journey has revealed a pattern. With every diagnosis, every flare, every crisis, I would hear that voice, that question playing over and over like a broken record. And with every episode, God took the opportunity to answer me. When I cried out to Him in the wee hours, alone in a hospital room, He filled the room with His unmistakable presence. My tears changed from frustrated ones to tears of relief and awe that God heard and visited me in a way that I could recognize. It is always amazing how just knowing He is near is enough to change everything. His very presence drives out fear and panic, and brings a flood of peace that can carry you through anything.

I believe that we become so consumed with our everyday obligations that we forget to seek God. Sure, we pray when we need something, return thanks for meals, maybe even spend time in daily devotions. But, we don't generally seek God just because we desire His nearness. In a romantic relationship, people tend to look for any opportunity to call or spend time with their significant others. And when they receive their call, they tend to stop whatever they are doing, if only momentarily, to acknowledge them and find out the reason for the call. How would it affect our relationships with God, and ultimately our lives, if we took the time to seek Him, just because we want to be close to Him?

The more time we spend with Him, the closer we become, and the more aware we are of His constant presence. He desires this intimacy with us so that doubt cannot gain any ground with us, even in the most unfavorable conditions. When we reach out for

Him on a regular basis, we can approach adversity with even more confidence. That is not to say that you will never feel lonely or that you will never be afraid—those are perfectly natural reactions to difficult situations. But, when that little voice begins to ask, "Where is God?", you can answer honestly from a place of experience, "God is here, with me always".

The Bible says that "faith is the substance of things hoped for, the evidence of things not seen" (Hebrews 11:1, KJV). The Contemporary English Version says it this way: "Faith makes us sure of what we hope for and gives us proof of what we cannot see." Where does the Believer's hope come from? Jeremiah spoke about hope in Lamentations 3. The prophet went into great detail about his persecution and hardship, but his conclusion was that through it all, he maintained hope because he remembered how great God's mercy is and that He had never failed to show His compassion. When you find yourself feeling out of touch with God or you are having trouble sensing His nearness and feeling His love, think back to how God has taken care of you all along. Think about the miracles you've witnessed, big or small, that only God could have done, and the ways that only He could have made. Even though you may not know His plan and cannot understand His will, God's track record of coming through for you in the past should be enough for you to extend to Him a line of credit, so to speak, that you can accept His promises as fact, despite how your current situation appears.

Each time we face a struggle and God brings us through it, our faith increases and the voices of fear and doubt become fainter.

Soon, we will no longer need to rely on what we've read, been taught or heard in someone else's testimony. We begin to know, really *know*, for ourselves, that no matter what condition or predicament we are in, God is right there with us.

Chapter Five: MISINTERPRETATIONS OF FAITH

I have undergone a number of physical changes since being diagnosed with lupus. When others first start to notice, they tend to ask a lot of questions. Their motives for asking are varied. Some are genuinely concerned for my well-being. Some ask because my symptoms seem familiar to them. Some ask because they plan to use the information against me somehow. And some people are just plain nosy.

Often, the most difficult ones to deal with, however, are the well-meaning Christians who want to use your situation as an opportunity to exercise their faith. You know the type—the ones who visit you at the hospital and pray for God to "raise you up according to your faith", or they tell you that they aren't "claiming your sickness". When you describe your symptoms or explain the diagnosis they tell you not to "speak it".

I have faith, too, and I believe that God is a Healer. I know that He is not the author of sickness or pain, and that He desires for us to prosper and be healthy (III John 1:2). But, I don't think that illness is the result of lack of faith. I know that death and life are in the power of the tongue. But there is a vast difference between "speaking things that be not" and acknowledging things that already "be" (pardon my grammar).

Accepting a condition enables you to deal with it—to find effective and productive ways to progress through life. Some people feel that by "claiming" or acknowledging a medical condition, that you are not trusting God to be able to change it--

that, somehow, by calling it by name that you authorize its presence in your life. But, the Bible describes Job as an exemplary man of faith and says that God had great confidence in him. Yet, he was faced with a serious medical condition because the devil was *allowed* to test him (Job 1:12). A medical diagnosis represents the existence of something foreign happening in your body. I believe that it is important to acknowledge that nothing can happen to us except that God allows it. And if He allows it, He knows that it is there. Thus, not "claiming" it is not so much an indication of faith as it is an indication of denial.

When someone refuses to acknowledge a sickness, it may appear that he or she does not believe that God can overcome something that can be identified—that He can only deal in the ambiguous and the obscure. Or is it that we feel the need to leave God some wiggle room, just in case things don't turn out the way we think they should? It's as if people think that if they don't call it by its diagnosis, then they are leaving God a loophole, in case He doesn't heal them.

I have seen God heal people with all sorts of ailments, repair body parts that doctors said would never work again and miraculously disprove all the empirical evidence that the medical professionals had to substantiate their findings. I have seen people outlive the most optimistic life expectancy assigned to them by the experts. I've seen tumors disappear and surgeries cancelled. The doctors do not have the final say, under any circumstance.

Acknowledgement of a condition—even calling it by name—doesn't give it any new fuel or authority. In fact, identifying it and then seeing God eliminate it brings even more glory to Him. When an x-ray shows a tumor, and a biopsy confirms its malignancy, and then it disappears the day before surgery is scheduled to remove it, that makes a lasting impact on everyone involved. When every known treatment has been tried and none of them works, then the patient returns to the doctor without a single symptom, the hand of God has to be acknowledged. God chooses to heal, or not heal, in His own time. It is counterproductive to question Him or try to rush Him. His will is always perfect, and His timing is never off.

If I can be completely honest with you, I am easily frustrated by those who wish to lay hands on me and demand God's healing. Some Christians think that if you don't pray for healing it Is because you don't believe, and if you don't get healed after receiving prayer, it is because your faith is inadequate. I submit that it usually takes more faith to accept one's condition with grace than it does to keep begging God to take it away. Anyone can trust a God Who never allows sickness to touch their life. But it requires a deeper faith and a genuine relationship with God to know that He is still an omnipotent, omniscient, loving and faithful God, even when He allows the things we would never have chosen for ourselves. It has been during this experience that I have seen firsthand His love, concern and compassion for me. He has been very present in the best and worst of times—often manifesting His love through the actions of people.

Since the lupus flare that landed me in the hospital for sixteen days, recurrent muscle spasms have prohibited me from driving.

At first, I thought that would be impossible to deal with, but God's faithfulness became evident in the willingness of others to provide whatever transportation I need. The loss of wages during my hospitalization and recovery imposed a great financial strain, but somehow, God took my "not enough" and not only sustained me, but even allowed me to share with others. When I shouldn't have been able to make ends meet, He was my Provider. When I was physically vulnerable, He protected me. When I was lonely, He comforted me. Many times, I would get random phone calls, cards or visits. And I cannot tell you enough about the blessing of my unexpected friends—those "angels" on Earth that God uses to remind us of His ever-present love and mindfulness toward us.

Certainly, God is a Healer, but He can still bless me and use me in spite of my physical condition. I will continue to worship and trust Him in the face of it. If he never takes it away, if the pain gets worse, if I lose all I have, He is still able, He is still worthy and, He is still God. **My experience feeds my faith when my circumstances do not support what I believe.**

MISERABLE COMFORTERS

An infuriating misconception that many well-intentioned believers have is that sickness is a form of punishment that God uses to get us "in line". It is hurtful when someone you care about is under the impression that something you have or have not done has angered God so much that He would strike you with illness.

Our God is loving, and satisfies us with good things. He is Jehovah Rapha—by nature, He is *Healing* itself. How angry would He have to be at His own child, a Believer, that he would deny His very nature and afflict them willfully?

The Biblical account of the story of Job tells us that He was one of God's faithful followers. So faithful, in fact, that when the devil doubted that anyone could have that much faith, God recommended Job as an example. He gave the devil permission to do anything to Job, short of killing him. In addition to becoming sick, Job lost his entire family and all of his wealth. This is not the only instance in which someone in the Bible endured sickness so that God's glory could be revealed. Even so, God was not the author of the affliction. When it was over, God rewarded Job for his faith by giving him twice as much as he had before.

When Job's friends visited him, they assumed that he had somehow brought his suffering upon himself. He referred to them as "miserable comforters" (Job 16:2). You may have similar experiences where a friend's visit or phone call may leave you feeling worse than you did before you talked to them, because they have somehow blamed you for your own condition.

Even in the New Testament, Jesus allowed Lazarus (John 11:1-44) and Jairus' daughter (Luke 8:40-56), among others, to die, and then proved that He is not only capable of healing, but that He is Resurrection and Life itself (John 11:25). If His goal had been punishment, there would have been some discussion of the healed person's offense—a moral to the story, so to speak—to teach us all a valuable lesson about the evils of their infraction.

Here is the reality—God is our loving Father Who wants nothing but good and perfect things for us. When He corrects or chastens us, He does so in love, just as we do with the children in our lives. No matter how big their mistakes or how badly they mess up, do we want to inflict harm on them? Certainly not. At times, discipline is necessary, and it tends to be unpleasant for both parties, but it is temporary and geared toward the teaching of a specific lesson. I don't know a single parent who would poison a child or purposely feed them something to which they are allergic, just because the child broke a rule, spilled the milk or came home late without calling.

We sin every day, and our mortal bodies simply could not handle the stress of enough sickness to punish everything we've done wrong. As Christians, if we believe that Christ died on the cross for our sins, why, then, would we tell a fellow Believer that God is punishing him or her? Perhaps we just have to face the fact that some people would rather accept a cruel and unlikely explanation than to admit that there are some things in life that we simply do not understand.

In the New Testament, the disciples inquired about an infirmed man, asking Jesus whose sin had led to his illness—his parents' or his own (John 9:2). Jesus informed them that neither was the case. I wish I could say that concept is an antiquated way of thinking, but I remember when AIDS and HIV became household terms in the late 1980's. Many ministers, televangelists, politicians, comedians and talk show hosts seemed convinced that this was God's way of judging homosexuals. Soon, it was understood that others had contracted the virus as well. Right or wrong, saint or sinner, God loves all of us, despite our hang-ups. According to II Peter 3:9, "it is not His will that anyone should perish". John 3:17 reminds us that Jesus came to save, not condemn. In fact, it's the devil's job to steal, kill and destroy, but Jesus came to make abundant life available to anyone who wants it (John 10:10).

The hope in that promise for us is that even a life with illness and pain can be rich and full. Because of the Christ, Who was wounded for our transgressions and bruised for our iniquities, and Whose stripes made perfect healing available to us, while sin can still *affect* us, it can no longer *infect* us. Accepting Him into your heart is the equivalent of taking a spiritual antibiotic. Sin that would manifest itself in the form of illness is warded off by the powerful presence of God's Spirit.

RESPONSE

How do you react when someone makes a judgmental comment that blames you for your condition? You don't. Reacting is an uncalculated, knee-jerk reply that does not leave room for you to process what has been said and what you should do with it. Before you give an answer, stop, think and then respond. It isn't instantaneous—it is a process. I recommend these steps.

1) SEPARATE yourself from the comment. You know that what was suggested is not the case, so becoming offended will require energy that the comment doesn't warrant. Refrain from replying out of hurt or anger just long enough to take step two.

2) CONSIDER the source. Whether the speaker is a traditionalist

who has been taught to believe that sin will make you sick, or some well-meaning soul who simply cannot accept the thought of not knowing the reason for such a serious condition, try not to react to the remark, but respond to the person.

3) PRAY for wisdom. "A soft answer turneth away wrath, but grievous words stir up anger" (Proverbs 15:1,KJV). Ask God for wisdom so that your response is informative rather than emotional.

4) EDUCATE. During your journey, you will disseminate a lot of information about your condition—to friends, family, employers, medical personnel, skycaps, waiters—the list goes on. Therefore, it is important to understand yourself—not just your physical condition, but do you know what you believe? I assure you, if you don't, someone else will be more than happy to tell you what you should believe. Unfortunately, they are not guaranteed to be correct. Examine yourself. Search your heart. Seek God. Do the research. Then, once you've spent some quiet time sorting through everything, live your convictions. I wish I could give you a formula or tell you how to answer a miserable comforter. But your response is most effective when borne out of a genuine relationship with God and a sincere and candid encounter with one's faith. Your reply can tell you (and others) where you stand in your faith journey. Check your attitude, and allow God to speak through you.

YOUR FAITH WILL MAKE YOU WHOLE

Okay, so maybe I'm not a theologian, but it just seems to me that there might be another interpretation of the New Testament instances when Jesus told people that their faith had made them whole. Certainly, they received a physical healing, but if that was His emphasis, I suggest that He might have said "Your faith has healed you", instead. The restoration of physical wellness does not constitute wholeness. I think Jesus was addressing the idea that when you have an encounter with the Christ and your faith connects with His power, He fixes *everything*: heart, mind, body and soul.

Perhaps the reason that our faith can make us whole and well is because healing has already been purchased for us back at Calvary. Because of the stripes He bore for us over two thousand years ago, healing already belongs to us when we accept Him as Lord of our life. To me, being "made whole" means being given the opportunity to "live one's life fully".

Maybe what the lepers and the woman with the issue of blood needed was to learn how to be whole, despite the damage their illness had done. These were people who had lost everything by the time they met Jesus. But their faith in the Christ and their contact with Him put them directly in touch with the God of all provision and health. The damage sustained by their bodies was the outwardly visible issue. The damage to their self-esteem, relationships and mental well-being were less apparent, but very possibly, even more critical. Before a person can undergo weight-loss surgery, he is required to go through counseling because of the mental and emotional adjustments they will have to make. His identity will completely change, they will see someone else in the mirror and people will automatically treat him differently than before. Sometimes people who have lost a lot of weight still wear oversized clothing because they still see themselves at their prior weight. I suspect the adjustment could be similar for someone who has gotten used to being sick and now has a brand new, healthy lifestyle.

Because Jesus' New Testament healings occurred before Calvary, they needed healing to be given to them. Healing is ours, but we still need to be made whole. That is where our faith comes in. Our God is the one thing that we can count on never to change— even when everything else is changing all around us. He is the solid Rock, and our faith anchors us to Him. Whether or not God heals you physically right away, you can, according to your faith, be whole.

Chapter Six: IDENTITY THEFT

If you allow it, your condition will begin to consume your time, your desires and, eventually, steal your identity. If you don't know who you are or what you are still capable of, you will become a victim of identity theft at the hands of your illness. This is usually the case when you begin to center your schedule, hobbies, grooming and relationships around a physical condition that is only one part of your life.

One way that I have started countering that is by not allowing lupus to be a reason for doing or not doing something. So instead of saying, "I don't cook as much as I'd like since I have lupus", I realize that lupus itself can't keep me from cooking, but my symptom management may dictate otherwise. Now, I might say, "I don't push myself to cook when I'm tired or hurting. But I still enjoy cooking when I feel rested". Instead of declining an invitation to go bowling with friends, because of the fibromyalgia pain, I might say, "I'd love to go along. Need a scorekeeper?"

It is a victory to celebrate your "can's" in the face of so many new "cannot's". And anything can be turned into a positive if you focus on the silver lining instead of the clouds. At one time, I had to receive monthly infusions. I spent a lot of time in my doctor's office in a leather recliner. I found, though, that the time flew when I started crocheting blankets for loved ones for the three hours that the IV delivered medicine to my body.

Sometimes, if I have difficulty sleeping, I convert the insomnia into thank-you time. I will think of someone who has been kind, influential or helpful to me, and write a brief note to them. By the time I've finished, I have been reminded of something very special, and have had the opportunity to let someone else know that they are appreciated. It is a brief distraction, and while it may not take the pain away, it does bring some pleasantness to help counteract the difficulty of the situation. When you can't sleep, or if you are in too much pain to do "standing" chores, pull up a chair to the kids' toy box and pull out some toys in good condition that could be a blessing to another child, a daycare center, or the nursery room at church. Closets and drawers can use the same attention from time to time, and when you are done, you will feel blessed to have been a blessing.

More than anything, doing something positive takes the focus off of the limitations that have recently changed your life. I believe that *you're not really living if you're not really giving*.

LOST

When you find yourself limited by your physical condition, it is easy to feel lost. You have invested time, energy, finances and emotional commitment into what you want to do and be. After all of your hard work, you have reached some of your goals and set your sights even higher—only, it seems, to have them dashed to the ground like a plate at a Greek wedding reception.

You've become known as the attorney, the engineer, the athlete, the entertainer, super-daughter or father-of-the-year. You've given your all to climb the ladder of success, and now, your body seems to have betrayed you, and you are forced to climb down backwards, rung by painful, depressing rung. Once you reach the bottom, there appears to be nowhere to go and nothing to do there.

When your self-image is shattered, often, your self-esteem goes with it. When you don't know what to do or who you are, you might be overwhelmed by a feeling of worthlessness. It is critical, here, to remember that you were always more than a title, a job description a relationship or a special skill. Every athlete, every musician, every professional is also a parent, a sibling, a son or daughter, a friend. Unfortunately, everyone cannot handle your situation, and relationships may change or end. You can choose not to break down just because your relationship broke up. Give yourself time to grieve over that loss, but then remember the ones who stayed. You will certainly find out who your friends are when your life turns upside down. Be thankful for the family and friends that remain in your corner, and be grateful that those who would impede your progress have removed themselves from the equation.

When you find that occupations or pastimes must change, keep in mind the other things that you still are. Focus on maximizing relationships, building new, forgotten or neglected skill sets, and enjoying other meaningful parts of your life. Spend more time with loved ones. Read those books or watch the movies you've been promising yourself you would "when you got the time". If you can't find who you are anymore, seek God's guidance. This may be your opportunity to re-invent yourself. Re-evaluate relationships, priorities and perspectives. Determine who you want to become and figure out the steps necessary to become that person.

The best advice I can give, though, is to take the lemons life seems to have handed you and make a lemon meringue pie or something. It starts with a decision. Within yourself, resist the urge to throw yourself a pity party. Make a conscious choice to think of others. If you like to cook, bake cookies with or for the special kids in your life. If you are going to a store, pick up a couple of things for an elderly neighbor or relative. If you aren't up to leaving the house, make a phone call to someone who isn't expecting it. Every day, tell someone that you love them. When others help you, say "thank you" and "please". You will be a blessing to many others, and I believe that blessings are like water—it's hard to splash someone else without getting some on yourself!

TURNING THE PAGE

For many, a diagnosis represents a new chapter in their lives. Too often, unfortunately, some tend to get stuck on the first page. But, reading it over and over again can make a single sentence seem like a *punitive* sentence. If you stay stuck on the "once upon a time", you will never get to the "happily ever after". Turning the page has nothing to do with forgetting. You will not forget the pain and/or symptoms you've been dealing with. You will not forget the fear you felt before your diagnosis. And you will not forget the sadness in your loved ones' faces when you shared the news. On the other hand, you also will not forget the joys of your past, the hope and prayers your family offered, or the strength with which you've overcome every other obstacle you've ever faced.

Turning the page simply means that you are ready to move past the initial emotions and reactions. Feelings of shock, fear, dismay and even anger are completely natural, but if you just marinate in it like a flank steak, you will miss out on all that life still has to offer. It is true that your everyday life will be peppered with challenges to overcome and adaptations to make. But you will also experience the joy of small victories and many unexpected pleasures and kindnesses. You will also come to know which friends and family members can be counted on, and be blessed by their stability and generosity. The condition itself may bring you into contact with great people. I have met doctors, nurses, techs and even maintenance workers whom I've never forgotten. They have impacted me with their kindness, sympathy, attention, wisdom, experience and information. This may not have been the ideal situation under which to meet them, but I am better for having encountered them.

My lupus flare was what daytime talk show hosts might call an "a-ha" moment. I'd like to think that I always cared about people, but never as much as when I was not able to do anything for myself. I was forced to depend on others, in pain, frustrated and scared. I gained new appreciation for those who were tending to me and tried to maintain a pleasant attitude. At the same time, I came to really understand that when someone else is facing adversity, their attitude and responses may reflect what they're feeling. I am learning to grant the same mercy and compassion that I have needed and may very well need again.

Not being able to drive for the last year has slowed me down. I spend more time with myself. The quiet is renewing—I can sort through all of the thoughts and emotions that I am often too busy to examine. I have time to commune with God. In addition, my family has shown such support that I've fallen in love with them all over again. I've had frequent muscle spasms that, at times, render me unable to control my muscles, so driving is out of the question for now. As much as I miss driving and my independence, I've enjoyed the time I spend with my dad, sisters, friends and godmother, driving to and from doctor appointments, tests, work or errands. It has been encouraging to learn how willing my co-workers have been in helping me get back and forth to work, and making sure that social gatherings are accessible and comfortable for me. Knowing that they care enough to go out of their way just for me has been a gift for which I am beyond grateful.

There will always be challenges, tough days and thoughtless people. But once you've read that page, turn it and find out what happens next in the story. If you keep re-reading that page, you may miss something wonderful.

Chapter Seven: TOUGH LOVE

Hurting and being sick is not fun, and you certainly don't need anyone to make you feel worse. But there are some things that you need to know that don't need to be sugar-coated.

1) **You are not the first person to go through this.** No matter how bad you feel, there are thousands of people who feel a lot worse. Feeling sorry for yourself does not accomplish anything, and certainly will not make you feel better. In fact, while no one expects you to sing and dance your way through life, be mindful that your loved ones have challenges, too. Your friends and family will probably listen to you vent and are even genuinely interested in your well-being. But no one wants to listen to a broken record.

2) **The doctors can only do so much—you *must* participate in your own treatment.** While you may be used to new symptoms cropping up every day, they may not be as random as they might seem. Your physician needs to know all of these things in order to observe any patterns. These may prove to be indicative of something else. A symptom that you usually dismiss may actually be a side effect of a new medication, or something potentially more serious. Follow your doctor's treatment plan. If the medication makes you feel funny, call the doctor—don't just stop taking it. If you are supposed to eliminate certain things from your diet, follow instructions. Ignoring your dietary restrictions may not produce immediate

symptoms, but you may be doing long-term damage. Note or document changes—when symptoms improve or worsen, keep track so that you will learn what works and what does not. Be as diligent with managing your illness as you are with your kids, job or ministry. It honors God when we do what we know to be right—in every circumstance. Your health is no exception.

3) **Don't make yourself your only focus.** When you don't feel well, it is easy to dwell on your needs. Don't forget, however, that the ones who meet your needs also have needs of their own. Be considerate. When you ask how someone is doing, really pay attention to their answer, and respond with compassion and sensitivity. If you require assistance, make it as easy and pleasant as possible for your helper. Every time someone does something for us, it requires time and resources that they could use for themselves. Genuinely express gratitude *every* time. Don't take anyone's kindness for granted. Reciprocate where you can—it may not be the exact same way, but the concern will be. No matter what, ALWAYS say "thank you"—it goes a very long way.

4) **Who are you trying to impress?** I know that you want to do everything you've always done. You want to maintain as much normalcy as possible in your daily life. But as honorable as it is to keep your commitments and not let others down, there *will* be some times when people ask for your help and you will have to say "no". Maybe someone will be disappointed, but the reality is that chronic pain/illness may require some selfishness from

time to time because other people only know what they want and sometimes have no concept whatsoever of what *you* need. It doesn't serve anyone's cause for you to overextend yourself. This will only put you out of commission, and leave you unable to help anyone, including yourself. Take care of yourself so that you can take care of others.

5) **Work smarter, not harder.** There will always be things that need to get done. But completing everyday tasks may be more challenging than in the past. Focus on making realistic goals. It can be very discouraging to bite off more than you can chew. Take the pressure off of yourself to do more than you are physically able. If you don't feel like vacuuming the floor this morning, I guarantee the lint will still be on the floor this afternoon after you take a nap. My mail comes in through a slot in my front door, so it lands on the floor in the entry way. I don't feel pressured anymore to pick it up immediately. No one else is affected by it, and there is no prize given if I do it right away. Pushing yourself when you're already weak or in pain will leave you feeling worse than you did when you started. Give your body a chance to regroup or recuperate before demanding it to perform.

6) **Stop postponing your life until you feel better.** A lot of people who are dieting wait to purchase new clothes until they have reached their goal weight. It is unfortunate, however, that they spend a lot of time wearing clothes that are ill-fitting because they have already lost some weight. But not dressing for one's current body type does

nothing for their self-image, but rather, reinforces feelings of inadequacy, instead of celebrating the progress they have already made.

A lot of chronic illness/pain patients tend to press the "pause" button on their lives. They put their goals on hold, postpone major events, even avoid relationships until they "feel" better or "more like themselves". But there is no way to know when that might happen. Certainly, if your symptoms limit you physically, there may be only so much you can do. But every day should see you taking a step toward your goal. A writer who creates only one sentence per day will have made a significant accomplishment after just a year. Crochet one row of an afghan per day and it can be completed in a few short months. Rather than feeling incapable and doing nothing, you will be able to celebrate your progress and be proud of what you have to show for your time.

Perhaps you are hesitant to begin a new friendship relationship, because you don't want to take that person through the roller coaster of your condition. Often, it is because you are afraid of being rejected if they decide that your needs are too great. But I have learned that some people are wired to be able to help you handle whatever you have to endure. God knows exactly what you need, and resisting their involvement in your life will cause you to miss out on the genuine concern and thoughtfulness that He designed to strengthen and encourage you. I can only imagine how much harder my recovery would have been without the people God has sent my way.

Embrace life. Carpe diem—seize the day! Find ways to enjoy every moment, despite the pain. You may be surprised how much easier it is to face tomorrow when you have genuinely enjoyed today.

Chapter Eight: THE COST OF LIVING

Making ends meet can be hard enough for someone who is perfectly healthy. So for those of us with special health concerns, the challenge becomes even greater. Just staying alive can cost you an arm and a leg! There are appointments to make, prescriptions to fill and exorbitant bills to pay. Getting and staying well is anything but affordable. And, at times, it can be tempting to cut corners when it comes to your health, especially when the air conditioner goes out at the beginning of the summer or your car breaks down in the middle of nowhere. I understand the immediacy of some needs versus others, but I implore you to consider this. Once you allow your health to deteriorate to a certain degree, it is very difficult to recover. Most chronic illness patients will experience peaks and valleys anyway, so it is imperative that we do all we can to stay in the best condition possible, so that the next episode doesn't take such a toll on our bodies.

In the interest of staying well, we must give ourselves permission to be aware of our value to God. Everyday, He invests in us life, resources, love and attention, and I believe that He is expecting a return on that investment. Simply put, if He allows us to be here, it is because He has a purpose for us, and we have a responsibility to pursue and fulfill it. We are admonished in Romans 12:1 to present our bodies as a living sacrifice to God, which is considered a form of worship. The condition in which we keep our bodies should be a testament to how we feel about Him.

If God believes in us so much that He compensates for whatever is wrong in our bodies just to keep us alive, how much, then, should we value our own lives and seek to maximize our experiences? And when we don't do all we should for ourselves, healthwise, what does that say to God about how we feel regarding the bodies He loaned to us? If you are someone who skips doses of medications frequently to save money or cancels doctor visits or refuses to go to the emergency room when necessary just to avoid the co-pay, I challenge you to consider the value God places on your life and then re-examine your attitude towards your health care.

Every penny you spend on getting or staying well should be seen as an investment in becoming what God wants you to be. You are not your own, but were purchased at Calvary. God has a plan for your life, and redeemed on purpose, for a purpose. So, then, we are obligated to take care of our bodies and do something productive with them. I know that even quality foods, like fresh produce and lean proteins can be expensive. Fast food dollar menus are much more convenient and affordable, but the food they offer, in large quantities over time, will kill us slowly. So what do we do?

Hobbyists, sports enthusiasts and collectors tend to be very passionate about their pastimes. There is no limit to the time, energy and money they will invest, because their hobbies bring them joy and satisfaction. By taking care of ourselves, we honor God, and enable ourselves to be around for our loved ones. We will miss out on fewer important milestones and occasions, make significant accomplishments and build strong relationships. Of all the things in life that we cannot control, managing our health care well is a choice that can make a lot of good things possible. Perhaps that is where we can find the joy and satisfaction that will make being well our passion.

Okay, money still doesn't grow on trees, right? And your finances are still limited. How can you afford to be healthy? It may require some sacrifice and creativity.

- Cutting corners is okay in some areas. On movie night, try renting a DVD from a vending kiosk instead of going to the theater. If you buy your lunch every day, try brown bagging it twice a week.
- Clip coupons for EVERYTHING!!! Check on-line for promo codes and specials—you'll be surprised what's available. Also, make use of the preferred customer cards or rewards programs. When you can, wait for sales, especially on big-ticket purchases. And when you go shopping, set a realistic budget and *stick to it!*
- Consider removing some features from your cable or satellite service. Decide if you can switch to a less expensive cell phone plan. Carpool to work or school to save on gas money.

If you've tried all of these suggestions, and there are just no more corners to cut, all is not lost.

- Communicate with your doctor. They can often provide free samples, discount cards and coupons for prescription meds.

- Ask your doctor if there is a generic form of the medicine being prescribed. They usually cost less than the name brand.
- Check with the pharmaceutical company directly. They frequently offer co-pay assistance for some drugs. I once was prescribed a drug that would have cost $11,125 out of pocket, per dose. After insurance, my co-pay would have been $125. After enrolling in their co-pay assistance program, I ended up paying nothing out of pocket.
- Check with your insurance company to see if they offer special programs related to your diagnosis. For example, my insurance company provides free diabetes testing supplies.
- Find the official organization that is dedicated to your diagnosis. Become a member and watch for updates, special offers and new treatment options. Always consult your doctor about whether these opportunities are appropriate for you.
- If you don't have insurance, check with local government agencies to see if there are health care programs for which you might be eligible. Also, some individual hospitals offer affordable health care options.

Making your health care affordable may require some effort, sacrifice, research and discipline on your part. But, remember, it is an investment in your own destiny, and a return on God's investment in you.

Chapter Nine: WHAT IF I DIE?

There. I said it.

While nobody really wants to think about it, the fact remains that no one lives forever. And while we'd like to think that we have access to an endless supply of tomorrows, if we are honest, we know that each of us has a date with our mortality.

So maybe the question we need to address is not "What if I die?", but "What if this condition causes me to die sooner than if I weren't affected by it?" There are several ways to answer this question. The spiritual answer is: "God's timing is perfect—even the time of our deaths". The philosophical answer might be: "There is no set time—death happens whenever and however it will". The medical answer may be: "There are so many combinations of factors affecting us at any given time that death is impossible to predict or prevent."

Ultimately, death has never been something that we could control. A diagnosis only makes us more conscious of death as a concrete reality rather than an abstract concept. In short, at some point, everyone dies. That is not the tragedy. I believe that it is infinitely more important to consider this question: "What if I don't live?"—not as a result of my illness, but because I neglect to enjoy my life to the fullest. *Do not allow yourself to become so afraid of dying, or so consumed with the challenges of your condition, that you stop living.* And don't be afraid to set goals or begin relationships because you don't know if you will be able to see them through. We are called to be good stewards of all that God has given us. *Time should be treated as an investment, not a formality.*

I have seen so many people become so preoccupied with the possibility of dying that they forget to focus on the certainty of the life that they do have. Their days become a series of doctor visits, hospital stays, medications, and symptoms—a mere existence. Their illness becomes the only focal point, reducing life to routinely going through the motions, when there is so much more. The people who love you will still want and need interaction with you. And no matter how self-conscious or frustrated you may feel, you need that contact with them as well.

Even if you make the most of every day you are blessed with, you may still wonder about and/or dread the effect that your absence will have on those you leave behind. It is important to realize that there is no way to avoid death when its time has come. The best we can do is to give loved ones the gift of our "best selves" now. Make your time with them quality time. In the end, they will be comforted by the type of memories of you that can bring you close with a single thought. And those who really love you will be most comforted by knowing that you maximized your experience. Whether one succumbs to illness, a freak accident or old age, the key is to live life fully, and without regrets. Instead of borrowing grief from tomorrow, allow today to be filled with the joy that God has made available to you. When your heart is full of God's love, peace and joy, there is no room for fear, dread or pessimism.

I have found several practices that consistently fill my heart and my emotional space with positivity.

- *Live life regret-free.* Make the best decisions you can with the information and resources that you have. Do the right thing for the right reason. Even if you make a bad call, there is no need to regret it because you made the best choice you could at the time.
- *Be kinder than necessary.* Kindness is not a competition in which you should try to outdo anyone. But it is also not something that you should withhold as punishment when someone does something that displeases you. Kindness is a gift to be offered freely. Know the power of kindness. Hold a door for someone. Greet people warmly. Make a gift of yourself—share the life that God has given you unselfishly.
- *Smile more.* It is very difficult to yell at someone while you are smiling. I have become aware of instances when I allowed stress to steal precious moments from my day. But I've learned that road rage does not make traffic move any faster. Profanity does not drive a point home any more efficiently than articulate speech. Arguments require more than one party. In these situations, make a decision to smile—it will give your brain a moment to redirect, and give your mouth a vacation from the instant negativity that can, unfortunately, become so automatic. Smiling during an argument may not always change the other person's mood, but it will take the edge off of your words, which can go a long way towards diffusing a

volatile situation. It will begin to come naturally if you allow smiling to become a habit. Besides, you never know who you will encounter that just needs to see a friendly face. Your smile just might make someone's day.

- *Be compassionate.* Everyone is dealing with their own issues. Try not to be so focused on your own that you forget the needs of others. If a waitress or cashier has an attitude, there is no need to flaunt one of your own. Instead, try putting yourself in their position—how many customers have complained today about things that were beyond their control? How long have they been on their feet today? And let's not even get into what they had to go through to even get to work or what they will face when they return home. Your understanding can go a long way to soothe that person, which may, in turn, yield an improvement in their service. Regardless, a word of encouragement or sincere patience may turn their entire day around, and you will have made the world a little bit better.
- *Love everybody.* You may not like them all, but treat people with love, no matter what. Walk a mile in other people's shoes. Offer comfort and understanding. Be considerate, and at times, choose to put others first, just because you can. They may never love you back, but if you sow seeds of love, you will, in time, enjoy a beautiful harvest.
- *Invest your time and energy.* Just as you would place your money where it can work best for you, spend your time on the things that will enrich your life. Friends, family,

dreams and goals must take precedence over worry, fear, depression and anger. There is only so much time in a day. Are you crying more than you are laughing? Are you worrying more than you are enjoying your loved ones? You will experience all of these emotions from time to time, but you decide what place to give them. Invest wisely and you will realize a greater return than you could ever have hoped for.

- *Be grateful.* I cannot emphasize enough how important this one is. When you approach life from a place of gratitude and humility, you will find that things that used to be so important will cease to matter. What was once critical will become inconsequential. You can find joy anywhere if you look for something to be grateful for rather than something to complain about. It may sound a little Pollyanna-ish, but there really is always something to be thankful for. Things really could be worse. Example: Instead of complaining, "I don't feel like going to work", you might remind yourself, "I am blessed to be employed" or "I am thankful that I am able to work". This gets me through a lot of days, and helps me not to dwell on the negative things that could easily pull my attitude (and subsequently, my quality of life) all the way under. Someone once said, "The best way to have what you want is to want what you have". The silver lining can be elusive at times. But make the effort to find it. It will be well worthwhile.

I suppose I didn't really address the question "What if I die?" very directly. I think that some things just have to take care of themselves. It is up to us to focus on the things that we can change or control. Forget about the ending, and look at all the potential new beginnings. Challenge yourself to take ownership of your life and your time. Experience everything to the fullest. Appreciate everyone. Meditate on the saying "Today is a gift— that's why it's called the present". Start asking yourself: WHAT IF I LIVE?! And then, go out and do it!

Chapter Ten: THE MINDSET OF A CHAMPION

Championships, in any sport or game, are considered to be the ultimate measure of a team or competitor's skill. It is not enough to win or be the best once—that could prove to be a fluke, because any number of factors could have an influence on the game's outcome. A tailwind, a pre-game argument, a migraine, even a really loud sneeze from a spectator can be the difference between victory and defeat.

Often, in order to earn the title of "champion", a team or competitor must triumph throughout a tournament. The tournament consists of several matches or rounds of competition, held under comparable circumstances. The idea is to determine whether there is one "best" overall. Those who are defeated are eliminated in the preliminary rounds. Those who are prepared, conditioned and focused, theoretically, will emerge victorious through round after round of competition.

But championships are not won all at once. The competitors who consistently win are the ones who concentrate on one game at a time. No matter how crushing your last victory was or how intimidating your next opponent is, none of it matters if you don't give your best in today's contest. Certainly, winners learn from each experience, but dwelling on the past can diminish future opportunities. If you are constantly looking behind you, how can you ever possibly prepare for what is ahead?

Just as tournaments are won one game at a time, each game is won one play at a time. Every chess player thinks ahead several moves. He is careful to ensure that his piece winds up in a favorable position, without giving his opponent any advantage in the process. A tennis player's serve dictates a lot about her opponent's return. A lot of strategic thought goes into how she aims. Even in figure skating, the athlete knows at the beginning of the routine how much speed is required to successfully complete a jump or how wide an arc to skate in order to end up in the right place at the right time. The key is that each competitor must focus on each move in succession. The chess player's bishop may be captured. Since he cannot get it back, he must shake off the loss and focus on how to use the next move to protect the queen. The tennis player's opponent may not return the serve at all, but she still must look ahead to the next play. And the figure skater may fall or stick the landing, but either way, there is another jump coming up in the routine, and the judges are still keeping score. Each has a desired overall outcome, but must narrow his focus throughout, in order to realize the greater goal.

Every NFL team wants to win the Superbowl championship, but none of them can win it in August. They must show up and play all season. There may be some losses during the regular season, but they do not give up because a loss does not necessarily make them ineligible for the playoffs. I know it can be hard to deal with a chronic condition, day after day, symptom after symptom, but you must summon your inner champion, and keep suiting up and giving your all on the field. When we show up for the game, it means we are ready to follow doctor's orders, be consistent with treatment regimens and dietary requirements. It means getting the proper rest and seeking the necessary support. Sometimes, it means doing our own research so that we can have a better understanding of what's happening in our bodies. And of course, it means having the best attitude possible towards what we are facing, and being able to make mental adjustments when we face challenges or become frustrated or tired. Most of all, it means that we must nurture our relationship with God, and look to Him for guidance, comfort, hope and wisdom. It is difficult to play sometimes, but remember, each season (flare, relapse, episode, crisis) only lasts for a set time, and then we can look forward to an off-season with fewer challenges. Until then, we just have to keep suiting up and taking the field.

One of the main reasons that taking each game one move at a time is so important is because a surprise move from the opponent may cause you to have to adjust your strategy. Flexibility is key, because if you become so committed to a single goal, you may miss an opportunity to advance or rebound. Football teams practice numerous plays so that they can change their strategy when necessary. This may require them to take a time out and regroup. As you play each game, keep in mind that you may, on occasion, need to take some time to re-evaluate your position, and possibly make some changes to your game plan. Consult with your teammates (family, medical professionals) and your Coach (God Himself) before deciding on your next move. I cannot emphasize enough that your condition is a process. It was not diagnosed overnight, probably didn't develop in a day, and you cannot expect to handle it, deal with it or "get over" it instantly. You will have to dissect, dismantle and reassemble it in your mind many ways before you will find *your* way of managing it. The thing to remember is to take things one day, one step, at a time.

Something in your environment or in your body has, in effect, declared war. And wars, my friends, are won one battle at a time (Oh, come on, you had to see that coming!). This point is critical to grasp because it is so easy to become overwhelmed when you are faced with a great big chronic diagnosis. It is natural to go into panic mode when someone says "NO CURE" and they're looking at you. But you can be the champion in this contest. Champions win because they keep returning, keep fighting and keep triumphing.

So, if this is a war or a competition, what is the prize? Well, that's up to you. You decide what you want. Your sanity, your goals, your family, your relationship, your future. You are fighting for control in your life—the right to put your condition in its place. If you walk into a barber shop or beauty salon without an appointment, you would expect to wait your turn until the stylist can make a place for you, right? The same goes for your diagnosis. It is an interrupter in your life, so it cannot unseat the things that are already part of your world. Certainly, your health is a great priority, but the illness itself is, if you will, "not the boss of you". I have decided that I have lupus, but I don't have to let it have me. I will not allow it to run my life or identify me. I accept the diagnosis and all of its implications, not as my destiny, but as a resource so that I can manage my condition in order to fully pursue being all of the other things that I am: a writer, a daughter, a sister, a friend, a Believer.

If you only remember one thing from this book, please remember this: "CHRONIC" is an adjective, nor a final ruling. It only has as much power as you give it, just like any other word. When I was in the first grade, there was an older girl who quickly decided that she didn't like me. Every day at recess, she would call me names. After trying everything I could think of to get her to stop, I asked my mother what to do. She said simply, "Just because she calls you something doesn't mean you have to answer to it. If someone has something to say to you, then she will call you by your name." The next day, the girl was at it again, following me around and calling me names. I was "smarty pants" by the monkey bars, and by the time I'd made it to the tether ball pole, I had graduated to "stupidhead". I kept quiet until, finally, she said, "Allison, do you hear me? Why aren't you saying anything?" I answered, "Because you didn't say my name, so you weren't talking to me." Of course, Mom was right, and her lesson has stayed with me. No one—the media, my employer, a doctor, or a friend—can tell me who I am unless I allow it. And just because they may try doesn't mean that I have to answer to what they call me. I am careful about calling myself a lupus "sufferer", become I do not want to give myself permission to become "one who suffers". That may be part of my condition, but it will not become who I am. I prefer to see myself as a warrior—prepared for a fight to the finish, one battle, one tactic at a time.

The Bible confirms this championship principle: "The race is not to the swift, nor the battle to the strong" (Ecclesiastes 9:11). Whatever your diagnosis, you are in control of your attitude towards it, and ultimately, how it will affect your whole life. Be sure that you define your condition instead of allowing it to define you. It is up to you to decide whether or not to give in and let your illness take over. The fight will become difficult at times, but a true champion is not victorious because the battles are easy. He triumphs because he keeps showing up and continues fighting, come what may. Even if you lose physical abilities, strength, or have to give up certain activities, as long as there is life, there is hope. As long as God allows you to be here, there is something that will make the effort worthwhile. Stay determined, and watch your inner champion emerge.

STRENGTH FOR THIS BATTLE

Once, during a lengthy hospital stay, a friend of my sister came to pray for me. The one thing I remember her praying for was "strength for *this* battle". It stood out to me, and I meditated on it for a long time. I appreciate her request more and more, because just like in a championship, I cannot afford to focus on what has happened in my medical history, nor what I may have to face in the future. When my condition challenges me and threatens to best me, my energy and focus have to be on the present battle. Certainly, I needed to concentrate on the symptoms I was experiencing at the time. But I also believe that every medical crisis is an opportunity for God to reveal something new or minister a reminder to me.

Spirits like loneliness, hopelessness, defeat and fear will show up. These are merely distractions intended to divert your attention from the place God has allowed you to be in. Romans 8:28 declares that "all things work together for [our] good…" That suggests to me, then, that God can use any and every part of a situation to change your life. I have come to realize that there are no coincidences—God has a plan for every experience you may endure, to make you better, to teach you, to draw you closer to Him, to help you make a transition.

Some of God's blessings are so subtle that they can be easy to miss, like an unexpected friend to go through a difficult time with you, or an opportunity to share your faith. I underwent a hemodialysis treatment that gave me a deeper appreciation for the intricacy of the body God has given me. I have so taken for granted the fact that my body worked properly. But spending time in an intensive care unit will quickly reveal how many people and machines can be necessary to monitor all of the systems that God gives function to every day in each of our bodies. When I went into kidney failure, I required so much attention that the nurses who took care of me were only assigned one other patient to look after. Yet, our God is so mindful of us, His precious creation, that He knows the number of hairs on our heads, personally counts our breaths, and composed the unique rhythm of each of our heartbeats. Even as we sleep, he keeps watch over us, giving instruction by His will, and life by His own power, and our bodies operate according to His commands. Surely, this God, my Creator, is able to sustain, repair and even re-create in me as He sees fit.

These encounters with God are the life-affirming moments that become "game-changers"—the moment in which we warriors begin to sense that victory is within reach. It is like getting a second wind that propels you toward the end zone, the basket, home plate or the finish line, just when you thought you were too battle-weary to last. These moments with God are the ones that win games and make champions of faith out of ordinary believers like you and me.

If we believe that God has a reason for every aspect of our journey, that He knows the plans He has for us (Jeremiah 29:11), then we should go into situations looking for Him, expecting to meet with His purpose. The last time I was in the hospital, my doctor made a decision that called for a procedure that needed to performed immediately. There was no time for family and friends to come and be with me for support. During this particular hospital stay, I had been having trouble finding God's purpose. But that day, when the door closed, and they were about to begin the procedure, I felt more alone than I can remember feeling in a long time, and God reminded me that He was with me. *"There will be some places along this journey,"* He spoke gently to my spirit, *"that no one can go with you but Me. But I am with you, always and everywhere. I will always be all that you need."*

Fear was defeated in that game-changing moment, and whatever worries I had about the procedure seemed to vanish. My faith caught its second wind, and I knew that I would be taking home another "win". I encourage you to seek God's purpose for every occurrence in your life, until it becomes a habit. I guarantee you, the more you look for Him, the more you will see Him.

Chapter Eleven: CHRONIC FAITH

Your condition is chronic.   But so is faith. People quote the scripture about how God can work with us even if our faith is as small as a mustard seed (Luke 17:6). Sometimes when we are faced with challenging situations, our mustard seed is a "mustered" seed, because we could only manage to gather the minutest amount of confidence. But the other side of the parable is that faith is a seed, and seeds grow. Perhaps instead of merely focusing on how little faith we are expected to have in the beginning, we should, at some point, treat it as if we expect it grow.

The mustard seed is an annual one—it is planted once and yields a harvest large enough that it will last until the next season of growth. Mustard seedlings emerge quickly and grow slowly. They require moisture and cold temperatures. These tiny seeds blossom into shrubs or trees, whose roots can grow five feet into the soil. When planted, the seed is only 1-3 millimeters, but the shrubs often reach heights of two to four feet. The seeds are harvested from a lovely yellow flower, and a delicious product is made from it and enjoyed by millions around the world.

Your faith should be the same. You may begin with just a little bit, based on what you've read in the Bible, learned in church, or witnessed from the lives of others. But when you plant it and allow it to grow, you can expect it to support you until the next growth season. The faith seedling bursts forth when the word of God clicks in your spirit, and you just "know" that what He says is true. It may be a small feeling at first—something that just makes you feel like you want to believe, even if you can't explain why. Faith does grow slowly—as you recognize God more and more as a present help throughout your life, not just in times of crisis, but you will see Him show up in everyday situations, reminding you that He is always near. These are the things that feed your faith. And as you water it with the word of God, it gains the nourishment it needs to sustain it, so that pests and harsh conditions cannot kill it off. Finally, it receives the light of the Son, which encourages growth.

Your faith requires lots of moisture—this may explain all of the storms you have had to endure. And faith thrives in cold temperatures. You may not have as many sunny days as you might prefer, and some periods may seem cold and lonely, but know that your faith roots are growing deep. In fact, the roots of your faith will grow even deeper than the part of you that you or others will be able to see. Isn't that the point of faith, though? That we will be able to have confidence beyond what we can see, touch or prove? Once your faith has matured, it will blossom into something beautiful that will not only be a blessing to you, but to all who come in contact with you.

I encourage you to be driven by your faith, not your circumstances. On your most difficult days, confront your condition with your confidence. Your illness and pain are not the last word—that belongs to God. In the midst of it all, I pray that you have encounters with God that will feed your faith, that you will embrace the hope of God's word, and that His peace and strength will accompany you along your journey. May you harvest an abundant crop of faith—enough to use and to share.

APPENDIX A: SIMPLIFYING YOUR HEALTH CARE MANAGEMENT

The following suggestions are intended to help you manage your health care as efficiently as possible. Adjustments may be necessary to suit your personal situation.

- Make a list of all doctors that you see regularly, what type of doctor they are, location of their office and their phone number. Be sure someone you trust has a copy or access to this list. Feel free to copy the form I use. (APPENDIX B)
- Maintain an updated list of medications you take regularly, and the dosages. Keep a copy with you—it can be difficult to remember details when you are in crisis. Include the name, location and phone number of your pharmacy. Also, note any allergies, both to food and drugs. (APPENDIX B)
- Keep a calendar of your appointments. Even if you always remember upcoming appointments, you may need to refer back to prior appointments.
- Note the dates of all surgeries, procedures, hospitalizations and special exams. (APPENDIX B)
- Write down new symptoms, concerns and questions prior to doctor visits.
- You may want to give your doctor's office the emergency contact information for someone you trust. This should be someone that you don't mind knowing details about your medical condition.

APPENDIX B: YOUR MEDICAL HISTORY

FULL NAME				DATE OF BIRTH	
DOCTOR	OFFICE LOCATION	PHONE NUMBER	TYPE OF DOCTOR		

DRUG	DOSAGE	FREQUENCY	PURPOSE
PHARMACY			
ALLERGIES			

SURGERY/PROCEDURE/EXAM/ HOSPITAL STAYS	LOCATION	DATE	RESULTS

www.ingramcontent.com/pod-product-compliance
Lightning Source LLC
Chambersburg PA
CBHW031300290426
44109CB00012B/652